Table Of Contents

Chapter 1: Introduction to Holistic Health and Wellness

Understanding Holistic Health

In today's fast-paced and demanding world, women often find themselves overwhelmed and struggling to prioritize their health and well-being. This subchapter titled "Understanding Holistic Health" aims to provide women with valuable insights into the concept of holistic health and its significance in achieving overall well-being and happiness.

Holistic health emphasizes the interconnectedness of the mind, body, and spirit, recognizing that true wellness cannot be achieved by focusing solely on one aspect. Instead, it encourages a balanced approach that encompasses various dimensions of life. By addressing physical, emotional, mental, and spiritual needs, women can experience a profound transformation and lead fulfilling lives.

When it comes to holistic health, it is essential to remember that each person is unique. What works for one individual may not work for another. This subchapter will introduce women to the idea of personalized guidance and support through health and wellness coaching. By working with a coach, women can receive tailored advice and assistance in achieving and maintaining a healthy lifestyle.

The subchapter will explore the benefits of health and wellness coaching, such as gaining clarity on personal goals, creating a customized action plan, and receiving ongoing support and accountability. Women will learn how coaching can empower them to make informed decisions, take charge of their health, and overcome obstacles that may hinder their progress.

Furthermore, this subchapter will delve into the various elements of holistic health that women should consider. It will cover topics such as nutrition and healthy eating habits, physical exercise and movement, stress management techniques, mindfulness and meditation practices, and fostering positive relationships and social connections.

By understanding the interconnectedness of these elements, women can cultivate a holistic approach to their well-being. They will learn how to nourish their bodies with nutritious foods, engage in regular physical activities that bring joy, manage stress effectively, and create a positive and supportive environment.

In conclusion, "Understanding Holistic Health" is a subchapter designed to introduce women to the concept of holistic health and the benefits of health and wellness coaching. It aims to empower women to take ownership of their well-being by providing personalized guidance and support. By adopting a holistic approach, women can achieve and maintain a healthy lifestyle that brings them happiness and fulfillment.

The Importance of Wellness for Women

In today's fast-paced and demanding world, prioritizing our overall well-being has become more crucial than ever, especially for women. Women play numerous roles in society - they are mothers, daughters, sisters, professionals, and caregivers, to name a few. Often, in the midst of fulfilling these various responsibilities, women tend to neglect their own health and well-being. However, it is essential for women to understand that prioritizing their wellness is not selfish; it is an act of self-care and self-preservation.

When we talk about wellness, we refer to a holistic approach that encompasses physical, mental, emotional, and spiritual well-being. It is about achieving a balance in all aspects of our lives, which ultimately leads to a happier and healthier existence. Women, in particular, face unique challenges and experiences that make their wellness journey distinct from men. Thus, it is important for women to recognize and address these specific needs.

Physical health is a crucial component of wellness for women. Regular exercise, a balanced diet, and adequate sleep are all essential for maintaining a healthy body. Regular physical activity not only helps in managing weight but also reduces the risk of chronic diseases such as heart disease, diabetes, and certain cancers. Moreover, a well-balanced diet provides the necessary nutrients for optimal bodily function and supports hormonal balance.

Mental and emotional well-being are equally important. Women often experience higher levels of stress and anxiety due to various factors such as work pressure, family responsibilities, and societal expectations. Incorporating stress management techniques like meditation, mindfulness, and self-care activities can greatly contribute to mental wellness. Additionally, seeking support from loved ones or professional counselors can be beneficial in managing emotional challenges.

Spiritual wellness focuses on nurturing our inner selves and finding meaning and purpose in life. Engaging in activities that align with our values, practicing gratitude, and exploring our spirituality can bring a sense of fulfillment and contentment.

As health and wellness coaches, our mission is to assist women in achieving and maintaining a healthy lifestyle through personalized guidance and support. By providing tailored strategies, we empower women to make informed choices that enhance their overall well-being. Through our coaching, women can gain a deeper understanding of their unique needs, develop healthy habits, and create a harmonious balance in their lives.

In conclusion, prioritizing wellness is not a luxury; it is a necessity for women. By taking care of ourselves, we can better fulfill our roles and responsibilities while living a more joyous and fulfilling life. Embracing a holistic approach to wellness, encompassing physical, mental, emotional, and spiritual well-being, can transform the way women experience life. So let us embark on this wellness journey together, empowering one another to live our best lives.

Chapter 2: The Fundamentals of Holistic Health

Nutrition and Healthy Eating Habits

In today's fast-paced world, women often find themselves juggling multiple responsibilities, leaving little time to prioritize their own health and well-being. However, it is crucial for women to understand the importance of nutrition and cultivate healthy eating habits to maintain a balanced lifestyle. This subchapter aims to empower women with the knowledge and guidance they need to make informed choices about their diet and ultimately achieve optimal health and happiness.

Proper nutrition forms the foundation of overall well-being. It not only fuels our bodies but also has a profound impact on our mental and emotional well-being. By adopting healthy eating habits, women can boost their energy levels, improve their mood, and enhance their overall quality of life.

One key aspect of healthy eating is the consumption of a well-balanced diet. This means incorporating a variety of nutrient-dense foods such as fruits, vegetables, whole grains, lean proteins, and healthy fats into our daily meals. Providing our bodies with a wide range of essential vitamins, minerals, and antioxidants helps strengthen our immune system, support healthy digestion, and prevent chronic diseases.

Another crucial factor to consider is portion control. Women often face societal pressures to adhere to strict body standards, leading to unhealthy relationships with food. Health and wellness coaches play a significant role in assisting women to develop a positive mindset towards food and encouraging mindful eating practices. By teaching portion control techniques and promoting intuitive eating, coaches can help women establish a healthy balance between nourishment and enjoyment.

Additionally, it is essential to address the common challenges faced by women when it comes to nutrition, such as emotional eating, stress-induced cravings, and time constraints. Health and wellness coaches can provide personalized guidance and support, helping women navigate these obstacles and develop effective strategies to overcome them. This may involve meal planning, stress management techniques, and incorporating self-care practices into daily routines.

By prioritizing nutrition and cultivating healthy eating habits, women can achieve and maintain a healthy lifestyle. The journey towards holistic health and happiness involves not only physical well-being but also nourishing the mind and soul. Through personalized guidance and support from health and wellness coaches, women can develop a positive relationship with food, gain a deeper understanding of their nutritional needs, and ultimately thrive in all aspects of their lives.

Physical Fitness and Exercise

In today's fast-paced world, women often find themselves juggling multiple responsibilities, leaving little time for self-care. However, prioritizing physical fitness and exercise is crucial for maintaining a healthy and balanced lifestyle. This subchapter aims to empower women to take charge of their well-being by incorporating regular exercise into their daily routines.

Exercise not only benefits our physical health but also has a profound impact on our mental and emotional well-being. It helps reduce stress, boosts mood, improves sleep quality, and enhances overall self-confidence. Moreover, regular exercise can prevent chronic diseases such as heart disease, diabetes, and certain types of cancer.

When it comes to physical fitness, it's essential to find activities that bring joy and fulfillment. The key is to create a sustainable exercise routine that suits individual preferences, abilities, and schedules. Some women may enjoy high-intensity workouts like running, kickboxing, or CrossFit, while others may prefer low-impact activities such as yoga, Pilates, or swimming.

Experimenting with different exercise modalities can help discover what resonates best with one's body and soul.

Integrating exercise into daily life doesn't have to be overwhelming. It can start with small steps, such as taking the stairs instead of the elevator, walking or biking instead of driving short distances, or engaging in active hobbies like gardening or dancing. Gradually, these small changes can lead to significant improvements in physical fitness and overall well-being.

For those who struggle with motivation or consistency, working with a health and wellness coach can provide personalized guidance and support. These professionals specialize in assisting clients in achieving and maintaining a healthy lifestyle. A wellness coach can help set realistic goals, develop a customized exercise plan, and provide accountability and encouragement along the way.

Remember, physical fitness and exercise are not about achieving a certain body shape or size; they are about nurturing and celebrating the incredible strength and capabilities of the female body. Embracing a holistic approach to health and happiness entails prioritizing self-care and making time for activities that nourish the mind, body, and spirit.

In conclusion, physical fitness and exercise are integral parts of a woman's journey towards holistic well-being. By incorporating regular exercise into our lives, we can experience improved physical health, enhanced mental and emotional well-being, and increased self-confidence. Whether it's engaging in high-intensity workouts or opting for low-impact activities, finding joy in movement is key. With the support of a health and wellness coach, women can create sustainable exercise routines that align with their unique needs and goals. So, let us embark on this empowering journey together, embracing the incredible strength and capabilities of our bodies.

Stress Management and Mindfulness

In today's fast-paced world, stress has become an inevitable part of our lives. As women, we often find ourselves juggling multiple roles and responsibilities, which can lead to overwhelming levels of stress. However, it is essential to prioritize our well-being and take proactive steps towards managing stress effectively. This subchapter explores the significance of stress management and the transformative power of mindfulness in enhancing our overall health and happiness.

Stress management is crucial for maintaining a healthy lifestyle and achieving holistic well-being. When left unchecked, chronic stress can have detrimental effects on our physical, emotional, and mental health. It can lead to various health issues, including heart disease, insomnia, anxiety, and depression. Therefore, it is essential to develop healthy coping mechanisms to combat stress effectively.

One highly effective approach to managing stress is mindfulness. Mindfulness is the practice of being fully present in the moment, without judgment. It involves paying attention to our thoughts, emotions, and sensations as they arise, allowing us to cultivate a sense of calm and inner peace. By incorporating mindfulness techniques into our daily lives, we can learn to manage stress more effectively and improve our overall well-being.

This subchapter explores various mindfulness practices that can help women in managing stress. It delves into techniques such as deep breathing exercises, meditation, and visualization, which can be easily incorporated into our busy schedules. Additionally, it provides personalized guidance and support to women looking to achieve a healthy lifestyle through the lens of health and wellness coaching.

Furthermore, this subchapter emphasizes the importance of self-care and self-compassion in stress management. It encourages women to prioritize their well-being and make time for activities that bring joy and relaxation. By nurturing ourselves and practicing self-care, we can build resilience to stress and enhance our overall happiness.

In conclusion, stress management and mindfulness are essential components of maintaining a healthy lifestyle. As women, it is crucial to prioritize our well-being and actively seek ways to manage stress effectively. This subchapter provides valuable insights, techniques, and personalized guidance to assist women in achieving a healthy and balanced life. By incorporating these practices into our daily routines, we can experience improved overall health and happiness.

Chapter 3: Assessing Your Current Health and Wellness

Evaluating Your Physical Health

As women, taking care of our physical health is essential for leading a happy and fulfilling life. In this subchapter, we will delve into the various aspects of evaluating your physical well-being and understanding how it can impact your overall wellness. By identifying key areas to assess and providing personalized guidance, you will be empowered to achieve and maintain a healthy lifestyle.

Physical health encompasses a range of factors, including nutrition, exercise, sleep, and regular check-ups. Evaluating each of these areas will enable you to gain a comprehensive understanding of your current state of well-being and make informed decisions to improve it.

Nutrition plays a vital role in our overall health. Assessing your eating habits, understanding the nutritional value of the food you consume, and identifying any deficiencies or excesses are crucial steps towards a balanced diet. We will explore different strategies to improve your relationship with food and develop healthy eating habits that will nourish your body and mind.

Regular physical activity is another key component of maintaining good health. Assessing your level of physical fitness, identifying areas for improvement, and setting realistic goals will help you create an exercise routine that suits your lifestyle and preferences. We will provide personalized guidance and support to help you make exercise a sustainable and enjoyable part of your daily life.

Sleep is often overlooked, but it plays a significant role in our overall well-being. Evaluating your sleep patterns, identifying any sleep disorders, and implementing strategies to improve the quality and quantity of your sleep will result in increased energy levels, improved mood, and enhanced cognitive function.

Lastly, regular check-ups and screenings are essential for early detection and prevention of potential health issues. We will guide you through the process of evaluating your current medical status, understanding the importance of preventive care, and establishing a relationship with healthcare professionals who can support you on your wellness journey.

By evaluating your physical health in these key areas, you will gain a holistic understanding of your well-being, enabling you to make informed choices and take proactive steps towards a healthier and happier life. Our personalized guidance and support will be invaluable in assisting you on this transformative journey. Remember, investing in your physical health is an investment in your overall well-being and happiness as a woman.

Assessing Your Emotional Well-being

In our fast-paced and demanding world, it is crucial for women to take a step back and evaluate their emotional well-being. Our emotions play a significant role in our overall health and happiness. By taking the time to assess our emotional well-being, we can identify areas that need improvement and take proactive steps towards achieving a healthier and more balanced life.

Understanding our emotions is the first step towards emotional well-being. It is essential to recognize and acknowledge our feelings, whether they are positive or negative. Many women often suppress their emotions, leading to increased stress and anxiety. By allowing ourselves to feel and express our emotions, we can begin to understand the root causes and work towards finding solutions.

One effective way to assess our emotional well-being is through journaling. Writing down our thoughts and feelings can provide clarity and insight into our emotional state. Take a few moments each day to reflect on your emotions, noting any patterns or recurring feelings. Are you experiencing joy and fulfillment, or are you feeling overwhelmed and dissatisfied? Being honest with ourselves in our journaling practice can help us gain a deeper understanding of our emotional landscape.

Additionally, seeking support from a health and wellness coach can be incredibly beneficial. These professionals specialize in assisting clients in achieving and maintaining a healthy lifestyle through personalized guidance and support. A health and wellness coach can help you assess your emotional well-being by asking thought-provoking questions, providing tools for self-reflection, and offering strategies to cope with stress and negative emotions. They can also help you set realistic goals and create an action plan to improve your emotional well-being.

Remember to prioritize self-care as you assess your emotional well-being. Engage in activities that bring you joy and relaxation, such as practicing mindfulness, engaging in physical exercise, or pursuing hobbies and interests. Taking care of your emotional well-being is not a selfish act; it is an essential component of overall wellness.

In conclusion, assessing your emotional well-being is a vital step towards achieving a healthier and happier life. By understanding and acknowledging your emotions, journaling, seeking support from a health and wellness coach, and prioritizing self-care, you can make significant strides in improving your emotional well-being. Remember, you deserve to live a life filled with emotional balance, fulfillment, and happiness.

Identifying Areas for Improvement

In our quest for holistic health and happiness, it is essential to take a step back and identify areas in our lives that could use improvement. This subchapter aims to assist women in recognizing these areas and providing guidance on how to make positive changes for a healthier and more fulfilling lifestyle.

As health and wellness coaches, our role is to guide and support our clients in achieving their personal goals. One of the first steps in this journey is identifying the areas that need attention. It could be anything from physical health, mental well-being, relationships, career, or self-care practices. By recognizing these areas, we can begin to develop a personalized plan for improvement.

When identifying areas for improvement, it is vital to adopt a non-judgmental and compassionate approach. Remember that we are all on unique journeys, and what may be an area of concern for one person may not be for another. Encourage clients to reflect on their lives and ask themselves what aspects they feel could use some attention or enhancement.

Physical health is often a significant aspect that women focus on. Encourage clients to assess their exercise routines, nutrition choices, and sleep patterns. Are there any areas where they feel they could make positive changes? Perhaps they need to incorporate more movement into their daily routine, improve their diet by adding more fruits and vegetables, or establish a consistent sleep schedule.

Mental well-being is equally crucial. Encourage clients to take stock of their stress levels, emotional health, and self-care practices. Are there any areas where they struggle? Are they taking care of their emotional and mental needs? It could be helpful to suggest mindfulness or meditation exercises, journaling, or seeking therapy as ways to improve mental well-being.

Relationships with others, including family, friends, and romantic partners, can significantly impact overall happiness. Encourage clients to assess these relationships and identify areas that may need attention. Are there any patterns of toxic behavior or communication breakdowns? Suggest strategies for effective communication, setting boundaries, and fostering healthy connections.

Lastly, remind clients to focus on self-care practices. Encourage them to evaluate how they prioritize their own needs and self-worth. Are they making time for activities they enjoy? Do they practice self-compassion and self-acceptance? Guide them in developing self-care routines that nourish their mind, body, and soul.

By identifying areas for improvement and developing personalized strategies to address them, women can embark on a journey towards holistic health and happiness. As health and wellness coaches, we play a crucial role in assisting clients in this transformative process, guiding them towards a healthier and more fulfilling lifestyle.

Chapter 4: Setting Goals for a Healthy Lifestyle

Defining Your Wellness Vision

In the journey towards holistic health and happiness, it is essential for women to have a clear vision of what wellness means to them. This subchapter will guide you through the process of defining your wellness vision, enabling you to embark on a personalized path towards achieving and maintaining a healthy lifestyle.

Your wellness vision serves as a compass, guiding you towards the life you desire. It encompasses all aspects of your well-being, including physical, mental, emotional, and spiritual health. By taking the time to define your wellness vision, you empower yourself to make conscious choices that align with your ultimate goals.

To begin, take a moment to reflect on what wellness means to you. Consider the activities, habits, and conditions that contribute to your overall well-being. Is it having a strong and fit body? Is it achieving a sense of inner peace and balance? Or is it finding fulfillment in your relationships and career? There is no right or wrong answer; your wellness vision is unique to you.

As a health and wellness coach, I encourage you to dig deeper and ask yourself why these aspects of wellness are important to you. Understanding your underlying motivations will help you stay committed to your wellness journey even when faced with challenges. It could be that you want to have abundant energy to keep up with your children, or that you aspire to inspire others to lead healthier lives. Whatever it may be, uncovering your "why" will fuel your determination and resilience.

Once you have a clear understanding of your wellness vision and the reasons behind it, it's time to translate it into actionable steps. Break down your vision into smaller, achievable goals that you can work towards. For example, if your vision is to have a strong and fit body, your goals could be to exercise for 30 minutes each day and incorporate more fruits and vegetables into your diet.

Remember, your wellness vision is not set in stone. It will evolve and adapt as you grow and change. Regularly revisit and reassess your vision to ensure it continues to align with your values, aspirations, and current circumstances.

In conclusion, defining your wellness vision is the first step in your journey towards holistic health and happiness. By understanding what wellness means to you, uncovering your motivations, and setting actionable goals, you pave the way for a fulfilling and vibrant life. Embrace the power of your wellness vision, and let it guide you towards a healthier, happier future.

Creating S.M.A.R.T Goals

Setting goals is an essential part of achieving success in any area of life, including our health and wellness. Without clear objectives, it can be challenging to stay motivated and track our progress. That's why it's crucial to create S.M.A.R.T goals – Specific, Measurable, Attainable, Relevant, and Time-Bound. In this subchapter, we will explore how to develop S.M.A.R.T goals that will help women in their journey towards holistic health and happiness.

Specific: When setting goals, it's essential to be specific about what you want to achieve. Instead of saying, "I want to be healthier," specify what that means for you. It could be, "I want to eat more fruits and vegetables," or "I want to reduce my stress levels by practicing mindfulness."

Measurable: Goals should be measurable so that you can track your progress. For example, if your goal is to exercise more, set a specific number of days or hours per week that you will commit to physical activity. This way, you can easily assess how well you are doing and make adjustments if needed.

Attainable: Goals should be realistic and attainable. It's important to set targets that challenge you but are within reach. For instance, if you currently don't exercise at all, setting a goal to run a marathon in a month might not be attainable. Start with smaller milestones, such as walking for 30 minutes three times a week, and gradually build up from there.

Relevant: Goals should be relevant to your overall health and wellness journey. Consider what areas of your life you want to improve and focus on goals that align with those aspirations. For example, if you want to improve your sleep quality, setting a goal to establish a consistent bedtime routine would be relevant.

Time-Bound: Goals need to have a timeframe attached to them to create a sense of urgency and accountability. Set deadlines for your goals to ensure you stay on track. For instance, if your goal is to lose 10 pounds, set a deadline of three months to achieve it.

By creating S.M.A.R.T goals, women can enhance their health and wellness journey. These goals provide clear direction, allow for effective tracking, and increase the likelihood of success. Remember, goals are not set in stone – they can be adjusted and modified as needed. Stay committed, be flexible, and celebrate your progress along the way. You've got this!

Breaking Down Goals into Action Steps

In our journey towards achieving holistic health and happiness, setting goals is an essential step. However, often we find ourselves overwhelmed by the enormity of our aspirations, unsure of how to proceed. That's where breaking down our goals into actionable steps becomes crucial. As women striving for a healthy lifestyle, it is important to approach our goals with a thoughtful and strategic mindset.

Breaking down our goals into action steps allows us to create a clear roadmap towards success. It helps us identify the necessary actions we need to take, making our journey more manageable and achievable. Whether you are aiming to improve your physical fitness, enhance your mental well-being, or cultivate healthier relationships, breaking down your goals will empower you to take charge of your life.

To start, it is essential to set SMART goals – Specific, Measurable, Achievable, Realistic, and Time-bound. Once you have defined your goals, it's time to break them down into smaller, actionable steps. This process helps you to analyze the bigger picture and identify the key milestones necessary for your success. By focusing on these smaller steps, you can make progress consistently, building momentum towards your ultimate objectives.

For instance, if your goal is to improve your physical fitness, your action steps could involve creating a workout schedule, researching and selecting appropriate exercises, setting aside time for regular physical activity, and tracking your progress. By breaking down your goal into these actionable steps, you can approach your fitness journey with intention and purpose.

As a health and wellness coach, you play a vital role in assisting clients to break down their goals into actionable steps. By providing personalized guidance and support, you can help women navigate through the complexities of their aspirations. Encourage them to identify the specific actions they need to take, create a timeline, and hold themselves accountable.

Remember, progress is not always linear, and setbacks may occur along the way. However, breaking down goals into action steps helps us stay focused and motivated, even during challenging times. It allows us to celebrate small victories and reassess our strategies when needed. By approaching our goals with a systematic approach, we can transform our lives and achieve lasting health and happiness.

In conclusion, breaking down goals into actionable steps is a fundamental process in our pursuit of holistic health and happiness. By setting SMART goals and identifying the necessary actions, we can create a roadmap towards success. As women aiming for a healthy lifestyle, breaking down our goals empowers us to take charge of our lives and make consistent progress. As a health and wellness coach, you have the opportunity to guide and support women in this transformative journey. Remember, breaking down goals into action steps is the key to unlocking our full potential and living a fulfilling life.

Chapter 5: Personalized Guidance for Optimal Well-being

Designing a Balanced Meal Plan

In today's fast-paced world, maintaining a healthy lifestyle can be a challenge, especially for women who are juggling multiple responsibilities. However, achieving and maintaining optimal health is crucial for overall well-being and happiness. One of the key elements in leading a healthy lifestyle is designing a balanced meal plan that provides the body with the essential nutrients it needs to function at its best.

When it comes to designing a balanced meal plan, it's essential to focus on nourishing the body with a variety of nutrient-dense foods. This means incorporating a mix of carbohydrates, proteins, and healthy fats into every meal. Carbohydrates, such as whole grains, fruits, and vegetables, provide the body with energy, while lean proteins, like chicken, fish, and legumes, support muscle growth and repair. Healthy fats, found in foods like avocados, nuts, and olive oil, are crucial for brain health and hormone regulation.

To ensure that your meal plan is personalized to your unique needs, it's important to work with a health and wellness coach. These professionals specialize in assisting clients in achieving and maintaining a healthy lifestyle through personalized guidance and support. They can help you identify your specific nutritional requirements, taking into account factors such as age, activity level, and any medical conditions you may have.

When designing a meal plan, it's also important to consider portion sizes. While it's tempting to indulge in larger portions, it's crucial to listen to your body's hunger and fullness cues. Opt for smaller, more frequent meals throughout the day to keep your energy levels stable and prevent overeating.

In addition to focusing on macronutrients, a balanced meal plan should also include a variety of micronutrients. These are essential vitamins and minerals that support various bodily functions. Incorporating a rainbow of fruits and vegetables into your meals ensures that you're getting a wide range of micronutrients.

Lastly, don't forget about hydration. Drinking an adequate amount of water throughout the day is vital for maintaining optimal health. Aim for at least eight glasses of water per day and limit sugary beverages.

Designing a balanced meal plan is a crucial step towards achieving and maintaining a healthy lifestyle. By working with a health and wellness coach, you can receive personalized guidance and support to create a plan that suits your unique needs. Remember to focus on nutrient-dense foods, portion control, and hydration, and you'll be well on your way to achieving holistic health and happiness.

Developing an Exercise Routine

In today's fast-paced world, prioritizing our health and well-being is more important than ever. As women, we often find ourselves juggling multiple responsibilities, leaving little time for self-care. However, establishing a regular exercise routine is crucial for achieving and maintaining a healthy lifestyle. With personalized guidance and support, we can create a workout plan that suits our individual needs, ensuring we achieve holistic health and happiness.

When it comes to developing an exercise routine, it's essential to consider our unique goals and preferences. Whether we aim to increase strength, improve flexibility, manage stress, or lose weight, there are countless options available. By working with a health and wellness coach, we can identify the activities that resonate with us and align with our desired outcomes.

One of the keys to success in developing an exercise routine is finding activities that we genuinely enjoy. This ensures that we remain motivated and committed in the long run. Perhaps we find solace in yoga, the perfect blend of physical activity and mental relaxation. Or maybe we prefer the invigorating intensity of high-intensity interval training (HIIT) to get our heart pumping. With the guidance of a coach, we can explore various forms of exercise and discover what sparks joy within us.

Furthermore, a holistic approach to exercise considers not only the physical but also the emotional and mental aspects of our well-being. Incorporating activities like meditation, mindfulness, or dance into our routine can help reduce stress, boost mood, and enhance our overall sense of well-being. A skilled health and wellness coach can introduce us to a range of practices that nurture our mind, body, and spirit, promoting a truly holistic approach to fitness.

Lastly, it's crucial to remember that consistency is key. Developing an exercise routine is a journey, not a destination. Starting small and gradually increasing intensity and duration can help prevent burnout and injury. With the personalized guidance and support of a health and wellness coach, we can establish realistic goals and create a sustainable schedule that fits seamlessly into our busy lives.

By developing an exercise routine tailored to our needs and preferences, we can achieve optimal health, happiness, and overall well-being. With the guidance and support of a health and wellness coach, women can embark on a journey towards holistic health, empowering themselves to prioritize self-care and make positive changes that last a lifetime. Remember, you deserve to thrive in every aspect of your life, and exercise is a fundamental pillar on that path.

Incorporating Self-Care Practices

In today's fast-paced world, women often find themselves juggling numerous responsibilities, from their careers to their families and everything in between.

It's no wonder that many women struggle to find time for themselves and prioritize their own well-being. However, self-care is not a luxury; it is an essential part of maintaining a healthy and happy lifestyle. In this subchapter, we will explore the importance of self-care practices and how women can incorporate them into their daily lives.

Self-care is all about nurturing your physical, emotional, and mental well-being. It involves taking deliberate actions to care for yourself, both physically and emotionally. As women, we often put the needs of others before our own, but neglecting our own well-being can lead to burnout and a decline in overall health. Incorporating self-care practices is not selfish; it is necessary for us to be our best selves and show up fully in all areas of our lives.

One of the first steps in incorporating self-care practices is recognizing the importance of self-care and giving yourself permission to prioritize your own needs. It's easy to get caught up in the hustle and bustle of life, but remember that you cannot pour from an empty cup. Taking care of yourself is not only beneficial for you but for those around you as well.

Next, it's important to identify self-care practices that resonate with you and align with your unique needs and preferences. This could include activities such as exercise, meditation, journaling, spending time in nature, or indulging in a hobby you enjoy. The key is to find activities that bring you joy and help you relax and recharge.

Once you have identified your self-care practices, it's crucial to schedule them into your daily or weekly routine. Treat these activities as non-negotiable appointments with yourself. Block out time in your calendar and commit to them just as you would any other important commitment. By making self-care a priority, you are sending a message to yourself and others that your well-being matters.

Additionally, seek support from a health and wellness coach who can assist you in creating a personalized self-care plan. A coach can provide guidance, accountability, and support as you navigate your self-care journey. They can help you set realistic goals, overcome obstacles, and stay motivated.

Remember, self-care is not a one-size-fits-all approach. It's about finding what works for you and incorporating it into your daily life. By prioritizing self-care practices, you are investing in your own well-being and happiness, ultimately leading to a more balanced and fulfilling life.

Chapter 6: Nurturing Your Mental and Emotional Health

Cultivating Self-Love and Acceptance

In our journey towards holistic health and happiness, one essential aspect that often gets overlooked is the practice of self-love and acceptance. As women, we often find ourselves striving for perfection, comparing ourselves to others, and feeling inadequate. However, it is through cultivating self-love and acceptance that we can truly embrace our uniqueness and live our best lives.

Self-love is not a selfish act but rather a necessary practice that allows us to develop a positive relationship with ourselves. It involves acknowledging our strengths, embracing our imperfections, and nurturing a deep sense of compassion towards ourselves. When we love ourselves unconditionally, we become better equipped to handle life's challenges and engage in healthy relationships with others.

Acceptance, on the other hand, is about embracing all aspects of ourselves, including our flaws and vulnerabilities. It is about acknowledging that we are perfectly imperfect beings and releasing the need for external validation. When we accept ourselves as we are, we free ourselves from the chains of comparison and create space for growth and self-improvement.

As health and wellness coaches, it is our mission to assist our clients in achieving and maintaining a healthy lifestyle. However, we understand that true wellness goes beyond physical fitness and nutrition. It encompasses mental, emotional, and spiritual well-being as well. By incorporating the practice of self-love and acceptance into our coaching approach, we can empower our clients to make lasting changes that extend far beyond the surface level.

To cultivate self-love and acceptance, we encourage our clients to start by practicing self-care. This includes engaging in activities that bring them joy, prioritizing rest and relaxation, and setting boundaries to protect their well-being. We also guide them in developing a positive self-talk and challenging negative beliefs that hinder their self-acceptance.

Furthermore, we encourage our clients to celebrate their achievements, big and small, and to practice gratitude for the abundance in their lives. By shifting their focus from what they lack to what they have, they can cultivate a mindset of abundance and foster a deep sense of self-worth.

In conclusion, the journey towards holistic health and happiness is incomplete without the cultivation of self-love and acceptance. As women, it is vital that we prioritize our well-being and embrace ourselves fully. By incorporating self-love and acceptance into our daily lives, we can unlock our true potential and live authentically, radiating joy and contentment. Let us embark on this journey together, supporting and empowering one another along the way.

Managing Stress and Anxiety

Stress and anxiety have become common companions in our fast-paced modern lives, and women often find themselves juggling multiple responsibilities, leaving little time for self-care. This subchapter aims to empower women with effective strategies to manage stress and anxiety, helping them achieve holistic health and happiness.

Understanding Stress and Anxiety

Stress is a natural response to demanding situations, but when it becomes overwhelming, it can have detrimental effects on our physical and mental well-being. Anxiety, on the other hand, is a persistent state of worry and fear that can interfere with daily life. Recognizing the signs and symptoms of stress and anxiety is the first step towards managing them effectively.

Identifying Personal Triggers

Each woman's experience with stress and anxiety is unique, so it is essential to identify personal triggers. Keeping a stress journal can help pinpoint specific situations, thoughts, or people that contribute to these negative emotions. By understanding these triggers, women can develop tailored strategies to manage stress and anxiety proactively.

Holistic Approaches to Stress Management

Holistic health and wellness coaching emphasizes a comprehensive approach to managing stress and anxiety. It encourages women to adopt healthy lifestyle practices that encompass physical, mental, and emotional well-being.

- Physical Well-being: Regular exercise, proper nutrition, and sufficient sleep are crucial in reducing stress and anxiety. Engaging in activities like yoga, meditation, or deep breathing exercises can also promote relaxation and a sense of calm.

- Mental Well-being: Cultivating a positive mindset, practicing self-compassion, and challenging negative thoughts are essential for managing stress and anxiety. Seeking professional help, such as therapy or counseling, can provide valuable support in developing coping mechanisms.

- Emotional Well-being: Nurturing emotional well-being involves finding healthy outlets for emotions, such as talking to a trusted friend or journaling. Engaging in activities that bring joy and practicing self-care rituals can also boost emotional resilience.

Building Resilience

Resilience is the ability to bounce back from adversity, and it plays a vital role in managing stress and anxiety. Women can build resilience through various techniques, such as setting realistic goals, cultivating a strong support network, and practicing self-compassion. Embracing a growth mindset and learning from challenging experiences can also foster resilience.

Creating a Balanced Lifestyle

In our pursuit of holistic health and happiness, it is crucial for women to create a balanced lifestyle. This means setting boundaries, prioritizing self-care, and making time for activities that bring fulfillment. By managing stress and anxiety effectively, women can cultivate a healthier and happier life.

Remember, managing stress and anxiety is an ongoing process that requires self-awareness, commitment, and practice. Through personalized guidance and support from health and wellness coaches, women can develop effective strategies to navigate life's challenges and embrace a more balanced and fulfilling existence.

Enhancing Emotional Resilience

In today's fast-paced and demanding world, it is essential for women to prioritize their emotional well-being. Emotional resilience, the ability to bounce back from setbacks and adapt to challenges, plays a crucial role in maintaining a healthy and happy lifestyle. In this subchapter, we will explore various strategies and techniques that can help women enhance their emotional resilience, enabling them to navigate life's ups and downs with grace and strength.

1. Cultivating Self-Awareness: The first step towards enhancing emotional resilience is to develop a deep understanding of oneself. By becoming aware of our emotions, thoughts, and reactions, we can better manage our responses to difficult situations. Self-reflection, journaling, and mindfulness practices can aid in this process, helping women gain insight into their emotional patterns and triggers.

2. Building a Supportive Network: Surrounding oneself with a supportive network of friends, family, and peers is vital for emotional resilience. Connecting with like-minded individuals who share similar health and wellness goals can provide a sense of belonging and support during challenging times. Engaging in group activities, attending wellness retreats, or seeking out health and wellness coaching can help women create and maintain this supportive network.

3. Practicing Self-Care: Self-care is not just a trendy buzzword; it is a crucial component of emotional resilience. Women need to prioritize their physical, mental, and emotional well-being by engaging in activities that bring them joy and relaxation. This could include exercise, meditation, pursuing hobbies, taking breaks, or seeking professional support when needed. By investing time and energy into self-care, women can replenish their emotional reserves and better cope with life's stressors.

4. Developing Coping Strategies: Life is full of challenges, and it is essential to develop healthy coping strategies to manage stress effectively. This may involve learning techniques such as deep breathing exercises, positive visualization, or mindfulness practices. Additionally, adopting a growth mindset and reframing negative thoughts into positive ones can help women build resilience and overcome obstacles with confidence.

5. Seeking Professional Guidance: Sometimes, enhancing emotional resilience requires professional support. Health and wellness coaching can provide personalized guidance and support to women in achieving and maintaining a healthy lifestyle. A wellness coach can help identify emotional challenges, set attainable goals, and create an action plan to enhance emotional resilience. They can also provide accountability and motivation, ensuring that women stay on track with their wellness journey.

By focusing on enhancing emotional resilience, women can empower themselves to face life's challenges head-on, maintaining a state of holistic health and happiness. Through self-awareness, a supportive network, self-care practices, coping strategies, and professional guidance, women can cultivate emotional resilience and truly thrive in all aspects of their lives.

Chapter 7: Building Supportive Relationships and Community

The Importance of Connection

In today's fast-paced world, filled with endless responsibilities and distractions, it's easy to lose sight of the importance of connection. As women dedicated to our health and wellness, we often focus on physical fitness and nutrition, neglecting the vital role that connection plays in achieving holistic health and happiness. In this subchapter, we will explore the profound impact that connection can have on our overall well-being and how it can be nurtured through personalized guidance and support.

Connection is a fundamental human need, yet it is often overlooked in our quest for wellness. As social creatures, we thrive on meaningful relationships and a sense of belonging. When we feel connected to others, we experience a deep sense of fulfillment and joy. Research has shown that strong social connections not only improve our mental and emotional well-being but also enhance our physical health. Loneliness and isolation, on the other hand, can lead to increased stress, depression, and a weakened immune system.

As health and wellness coaches, our role is not only to guide clients in making healthy choices but also to help them cultivate meaningful connections. We understand that true well-being is a balance of physical, mental, and social wellness. By prioritizing connection, we can empower our clients to develop a support network that will sustain them on their journey to optimal health.

Personalized guidance and support are key components of fostering connection. Each individual is unique, with different needs and preferences when it comes to social interactions. As coaches, we assist our clients in identifying the types of connections that align with their values and interests. Whether it is joining a fitness class, volunteering for a cause they are passionate about, or participating in support groups, we tailor our guidance to help them find the connections that will bring them the most fulfillment.

Furthermore, we provide ongoing support as our clients navigate the challenges and triumphs of building and maintaining connections. We offer a listening ear, encouragement, and practical strategies to overcome obstacles that may arise. Through our personalized approach, we empower women to cultivate deep and meaningful connections that enrich their lives and contribute to their overall well-being.

In conclusion, connection is a vital component of holistic health and happiness. As women dedicated to our wellness, we must recognize the importance of nurturing meaningful relationships and a sense of belonging. As health and wellness coaches, we play a crucial role in assisting our clients in achieving and maintaining a healthy lifestyle by providing personalized guidance and support. By prioritizing connection, we can help our clients experience the profound benefits that come from fostering authentic relationships and a strong support network.

Nurturing Healthy Relationships

In our journey towards holistic health and happiness, the importance of nurturing healthy relationships cannot be overstated. As women, we often find ourselves juggling numerous responsibilities, from careers to families, leaving little time for self-care and cultivating meaningful connections. However, investing in our relationships is crucial for our overall well-being and can greatly impact our mental, emotional, and physical health.

When we talk about nurturing healthy relationships, it goes beyond romantic partnerships. It encompasses our relationships with family, friends, colleagues, and even ourselves. These connections play a significant role in shaping our happiness and fulfillment, highlighting the need to prioritize them.

One key aspect of nurturing healthy relationships is effective communication. Clear and open communication allows us to express our needs, boundaries, and emotions effectively. It fosters understanding, trust, and empathy, enabling us to build deeper connections with those around us. As women, we often struggle to voice our feelings and set boundaries, fearing judgment or conflict. However, by practicing assertive communication, we can create healthier dynamics and cultivate more fulfilling relationships.

Another crucial element is self-care within relationships. It is essential to remember that we cannot pour from an empty cup. Prioritizing self-care allows us to show up fully for our loved ones while maintaining our own well-being. By setting aside time for self-reflection, relaxation, and pursuing our passions, we not only recharge ourselves but also inspire and uplift those around us. It is through self-care that we can truly nurture healthy relationships.

Furthermore, cultivating empathy and emotional intelligence is vital in fostering healthy connections. Empathy allows us to understand and validate the emotions of others, creating a safe space for vulnerability and growth. Emotional intelligence helps us navigate conflicts and challenges with grace, promoting understanding and resolution. By honing these skills, we can build stronger, more fulfilling relationships based on compassion and mutual support.

As health and wellness coaches, it is our responsibility to guide and support our clients in nurturing healthy relationships. By incorporating relationship-building techniques into our coaching practices, we can help our clients foster deeper connections, set healthier boundaries, and enhance their overall well-being. Through personalized guidance and support, we can empower women to prioritize their relationships and create a harmonious balance between their own needs and the needs of those they care about.

In conclusion, nurturing healthy relationships is an essential component of our holistic health and happiness. By practicing effective communication, prioritizing self-care, and cultivating empathy and emotional intelligence, we can create meaningful connections that enrich our lives. As women, let us embrace the power of healthy relationships and inspire others to do the same, fostering a community of empowered individuals who thrive in their personal connections.

Finding Supportive Communities

In the fast-paced and ever-changing world we live in, finding a supportive community can be a vital aspect of maintaining a healthy and balanced lifestyle. As women, we often juggle multiple roles and responsibilities, leaving little time for ourselves. However, nurturing our own well-being is essential for our overall health and happiness.

In this subchapter, we delve into the importance of finding supportive communities and how they can empower women on their journey towards holistic health and well-being. Whether you are seeking a support network to achieve your fitness goals, manage stress, or simply connect with like-minded individuals, joining a community that aligns with your values and aspirations can be transformative.

Health and wellness coaching plays a significant role in assisting women in achieving and maintaining a healthy lifestyle. The guidance and support of a coach can help navigate the challenges and obstacles that arise on the path to wellness. However, a coach can only provide individualized guidance for a limited amount of time. This is where supportive communities come into play.

By connecting with others who share similar goals and aspirations, women can build a network of support that extends beyond their coaching sessions. These communities provide a safe space to share experiences, seek advice, and celebrate achievements. They foster a sense of belonging and encouragement, creating an environment conducive to personal growth and empowerment.

In a supportive community, women can find inspiration, motivation, and accountability. They can exchange knowledge, resources, and strategies for maintaining a healthy lifestyle. Whether it's through online platforms, local meetups, or workshops, the opportunities to connect are endless.

Moreover, being part of a supportive community provides an avenue for women to explore and discover new avenues for self-care and well-being. It allows for the exploration of different modalities, such as meditation, yoga, mindfulness, and nutrition. By engaging with others who have similar interests, women can expand their horizons and find what resonates with them on their wellness journey.

In conclusion, finding supportive communities is crucial for every woman seeking to achieve and maintain a healthy lifestyle. By joining like-minded individuals on a similar path, women can find solace, inspiration, and guidance. These communities serve as a valuable resource, supplementing the support received from health and wellness coaching. Together, we can create a network of empowered women, supporting and uplifting one another on our quest for holistic health and happiness.

Chapter 8: Overcoming Challenges and Obstacles

Dealing with Setbacks and Plateaus

Introduction:

In our journey towards holistic health and happiness, setbacks and plateaus are inevitable. As women, we face numerous challenges that can often hinder our progress. This subchapter aims to provide guidance and support, specifically addressing the setbacks and plateaus that women may encounter on their path to achieving and maintaining a healthy lifestyle.

Understanding Setbacks:

Setbacks can come in various forms, such as unexpected life events, lack of motivation, or self-doubt. It is crucial to recognize that setbacks are a natural part of the process and should not be viewed as failures. Instead, they offer valuable learning opportunities. By acknowledging setbacks, we can better understand the underlying reasons and develop strategies to overcome them.

Overcoming Setbacks:

To overcome setbacks, it is important to cultivate resilience and self-compassion. Remember that setbacks do not define us; rather, they provide an opportunity for growth. By practicing self-compassion, we can treat ourselves with kindness, understanding that setbacks are part of being human. Surrounding ourselves with a supportive community, seeking guidance from a health and wellness coach, and creating a positive mindset are all crucial steps towards overcoming setbacks.

Navigating Plateaus:

Plateaus can be frustrating, especially when we feel like our progress has stalled. However, it is important to remember that plateaus are temporary and can be overcome with a shift in perspective and approach. Plateaus often occur when our bodies adapt to our current routines or when we become too comfortable with our lifestyle choices. To navigate plateaus successfully, it is crucial to embrace change and introduce new challenges into our wellness routines. This could include trying new exercises, exploring different approaches to nutrition, or seeking support from a health and wellness coach for personalized guidance.

Conclusion:

As women striving for holistic health and happiness, setbacks and plateaus are an inherent part of our journey. By understanding setbacks, cultivating resilience, and practicing self-compassion, we can overcome obstacles and continue moving forward. Navigating plateaus requires a willingness to embrace change and seek new challenges. Remember, setbacks and plateaus are opportunities for growth and self-discovery. With the right mindset and support, we can conquer any setback or plateau that comes our way, ultimately achieving and maintaining a healthy lifestyle that brings us joy and fulfillment.

Managing Time and Priorities

In today's fast-paced world, where women often find themselves juggling multiple roles and responsibilities, managing time and priorities has become more important than ever. As a woman, it is crucial to find a balance between work, family, self-care, and personal goals. This subchapter will provide valuable insights and strategies on how to effectively manage time and priorities, ensuring a healthy lifestyle and overall happiness.

One of the key factors in managing time and priorities is the ability to set clear goals. By defining what is truly important to you, you can create a roadmap for your life and make informed decisions about how to spend your time. Setting both short-term and long-term goals will help in prioritizing tasks and activities accordingly.

Another important aspect of time management is learning to say no. As women, we often feel obligated to take on more than we can handle, whether it be at work, home, or within our social circles. However, this can lead to burnout and neglecting our own needs. It is essential to establish boundaries and learn to say no when necessary, focusing on activities and commitments that align with our priorities.

Effective time management also involves creating a schedule or routine that works for you. This includes allocating specific time blocks for work, family, self-care, and personal goals. By establishing a structured routine, you can minimize distractions and make the most of your time. Additionally, incorporating time for self-care activities, such as exercise, meditation, or hobbies, is crucial for maintaining overall health and well-being.

To ensure efficient time management, it is essential to utilize tools and techniques that can help you stay organized. This can include using calendars, planners, or productivity apps to track deadlines, appointments, and tasks. By utilizing these tools, you can stay on top of your commitments and avoid last-minute rushes or missed deadlines.

Lastly, seeking support from a health and wellness coach can be immensely beneficial in managing time and priorities. A coach can provide personalized guidance and support, helping you navigate through challenges and develop effective strategies for balancing various aspects of your life. They can assist you in identifying your priorities, setting achievable goals, and holding you accountable for your actions.

In conclusion, managing time and priorities is a crucial skill for women seeking a healthy and fulfilling lifestyle. By setting clear goals, establishing boundaries, creating a structured routine, utilizing organizational tools, and seeking support from a health and wellness coach, women can effectively manage their time and priorities, leading to holistic health and happiness. Remember, time is a precious resource, and by managing it wisely, you can create a life you truly love.

Overcoming Emotional Blocks

In our journey towards a healthy and fulfilled life, it is essential to address our emotional well-being. Emotional blocks can hinder our progress and prevent us from achieving holistic health and happiness. These blocks may manifest in various ways, such as self-doubt, fear, anxiety, or even a lack of motivation. However, with the right mindset and strategies, we can overcome these obstacles and unlock our true potential.

Recognizing and acknowledging our emotional blocks is the first step towards overcoming them. As women, we often tend to prioritize the needs of others before our own, neglecting our own emotions in the process. However, it is crucial to give ourselves permission to feel and express our emotions without judgment. By doing so, we can begin to understand the root causes of our emotional blocks and work towards resolving them.

One effective way to overcome emotional blocks is through the practice of self-compassion. We often hold ourselves to high standards and beat ourselves up for not meeting them. However, self-compassion involves treating ourselves with kindness, understanding, and acceptance. It involves recognizing that we are human and that it is okay to make mistakes or experience setbacks. By cultivating self-compassion, we can learn to let go of self-limiting beliefs and embrace a more positive mindset.

Another powerful tool for overcoming emotional blocks is through self-reflection and journaling. Taking the time to reflect on our thoughts and emotions allows us to gain clarity and insight into our inner world. Journaling provides a safe space to explore our feelings, fears, and desires. It can help us identify patterns, triggers, and negative thought patterns that contribute to our emotional blocks. Through regular journaling, we can begin to reframe our thoughts, release emotional baggage, and create a more empowering narrative for ourselves.

Additionally, seeking support from a health and wellness coach can be immensely beneficial in overcoming emotional blocks. A coach provides personalized guidance, support, and accountability to help us navigate through our emotional challenges. They can help us explore our values, set meaningful goals, and develop strategies to overcome obstacles. With their expertise, we can gain valuable insights, learn new coping mechanisms, and cultivate resilience.

Overcoming emotional blocks is a journey that requires patience, self-compassion, and a willingness to grow. By addressing and working through our emotional barriers, we can unleash our true potential, achieve holistic health, and experience lasting happiness. Remember, you are worthy of living a life free from emotional blocks – embrace the journey and thrive!

Chapter 9: Maintaining Long-Term Wellness

Creating Sustainable Habits

In our fast-paced and ever-changing world, it's easy to get caught up in the chaos and neglect our own well-being. As women, we often prioritize the needs of others before our own, leaving little time and energy for self-care. However, by creating sustainable habits, we can reclaim our health and happiness, and become the best version of ourselves.

Sustainable habits are those that promote long-term well-being and can be maintained consistently over time. These habits encompass various aspects of our lives, including physical, mental, and emotional well-being. By incorporating these habits into our daily routine, we can gradually transform our lives and achieve holistic health.

One of the key aspects of creating sustainable habits is personalized guidance and support. As a health and wellness coach, my role is to assist you in identifying your unique needs and crafting a personalized plan that aligns with your goals. Together, we will explore various areas of your life, such as nutrition, exercise, stress management, and self-care, to develop a comprehensive approach to wellness.

In terms of nutrition, sustainable habits involve adopting a balanced and nourishing diet that provides essential nutrients for optimal health. We will work together to identify wholesome, nutritious foods that you enjoy and develop meal plans that are easy to prepare and fit into your lifestyle. By making small, gradual changes to your eating habits, we can create lasting and sustainable improvements to your overall well-being.

Physical activity is another crucial aspect of sustainable habits. Incorporating regular exercise into your routine not only improves your physical health but also boosts your mood and reduces stress. We will explore different types of exercise and find activities that you genuinely enjoy, making it easier to stick to a consistent routine.

Stress management and self-care are essential for maintaining a healthy lifestyle. We will explore various relaxation techniques, such as meditation, deep breathing exercises, and mindfulness practices, to help you manage stress effectively. Additionally, we will prioritize self-care activities that bring you joy and rejuvenation, such as taking a warm bath, reading a book, or spending time in nature.

Creating sustainable habits requires patience, commitment, and self-compassion. It's important to remember that change takes time, and setbacks are a natural part of the process. As your health and wellness coach, I will provide ongoing support and guidance to keep you motivated and accountable, ensuring that you stay on track towards achieving your goals.

By embracing sustainable habits, you can cultivate a lifestyle that promotes holistic health and happiness. Together, let's embark on this transformative journey towards a more fulfilling and balanced life.

Strategies for Staying Motivated

Introduction:
In this subchapter, we will explore effective strategies for staying motivated on your journey towards holistic health and happiness. As women, we often find ourselves pulled in multiple directions, and it can be challenging to maintain focus on our own well-being. However, with the right strategies and support, we can cultivate lasting motivation to achieve and maintain a healthy lifestyle.

1. Set Clear and Realistic Goals:
The first step towards staying motivated is to set clear and achievable goals. Take the time to reflect on what you want to accomplish in terms of your health and wellness. Break these goals down into smaller, actionable steps that

will make them more attainable. By having a clear roadmap and realistic expectations, you will feel more motivated to take consistent action.

2. Find Your Why:
Understanding your motivations and the deeper reasons behind your desire for a healthy lifestyle is crucial for staying motivated. Ask yourself why you want to improve your well-being. Is it to have more energy for your family? To feel confident in your own skin? Knowing your "why" will help you stay committed and focused, especially during challenging times.

3. Seek Professional Guidance:
Enlisting the support of a health and wellness coach can be invaluable in maintaining motivation. A coach can provide personalized guidance, support, and accountability to help you stay on track. They can help you create a personalized plan tailored to your unique needs, ensuring that you always have someone by your side cheering you on.

4. Celebrate Milestones and Progress:
Celebrate your achievements, no matter how small they may seem. Acknowledging your progress along the way will keep your motivation high. Reward yourself for reaching milestones, whether it's treating yourself to a relaxing massage, a new workout outfit, or a day of self-care. By recognizing your efforts, you'll build momentum and continue to be motivated.

5. Surround Yourself with Supportive People:
The company you keep plays a significant role in your motivation. Surround yourself with like-minded individuals who share your goals and values. Joining a community or finding an accountability partner can provide the encouragement and support you need during challenging times. Having someone to share your journey with makes it more enjoyable and significantly increases your chances of success.

Conclusion:
Staying motivated on your path to holistic health and happiness is essential.

By setting clear goals, understanding your motivations, seeking professional guidance, celebrating milestones, and surrounding yourself with supportive people, you can maintain your motivation and achieve a healthy lifestyle. Remember, motivation is not a one-time event; it is a journey. Embrace the process, be kind to yourself, and keep pushing forward. You've got this!

Celebrating Milestones and Successes

In the journey towards holistic health and happiness, it is crucial to acknowledge and celebrate the milestones and successes we achieve along the way. As women, we often prioritize taking care of others over ourselves, leaving little time to acknowledge our own accomplishments. However, it is essential to recognize and honor our achievements as they provide the motivation and inspiration to continue striving for a healthy and fulfilling life.

As health and wellness coaches, our role is to assist our clients in achieving and maintaining a healthy lifestyle through personalized guidance and support. Part of this process involves celebrating the milestones and successes our clients experience on their wellness journey. By acknowledging their progress, we empower our clients to recognize their own strength and capabilities, fostering a positive mindset that fuels further growth.

One way to celebrate milestones and successes is by setting achievable goals. Encourage your clients to establish small, attainable objectives that align with their overall wellness vision. When they reach these goals, celebrate their accomplishments with them. Whether it's losing a certain amount of weight, adopting a new exercise routine, or embracing a mindfulness practice, each milestone deserves recognition and applause.

Another effective way to celebrate milestones is through reflection and gratitude. Encourage your clients to regularly reflect on their progress and express gratitude for each step they've taken towards a healthier lifestyle. This practice promotes self-awareness and mindfulness, allowing clients to appreciate their achievements and the positive changes they have made in their lives.

Celebrating milestones and successes can also be a social event. Organize group gatherings or virtual meetups where clients can come together to share their achievements and support one another. This sense of community and camaraderie provides a supportive network that reinforces the importance of celebrating personal victories.

Finally, encourage your clients to treat themselves when they reach significant milestones. Whether it's indulging in a spa day, buying a new outfit, or taking a weekend getaway, these rewards can serve as a tangible reminder of their achievements. Self-care and self-love are integral to holistic health, and celebrating milestones is an opportunity to practice both.

In conclusion, celebrating milestones and successes is a vital aspect of the wellness journey. As health and wellness coaches, we play a crucial role in guiding our clients towards these achievements. By encouraging goal setting, reflection, gratitude, social connections, and self-rewards, we empower women to embrace and celebrate their progress, reinforcing their commitment to a healthy and fulfilling life. Let us not overlook the importance of these celebrations, for they serve as reminders of the incredible strength and resilience within each woman on their path to holistic health and happiness.

Chapter 10: Embracing Holistic Happiness

Finding Joy in Everyday Life

In our fast-paced and demanding world, it's easy to get caught up in the hustle and forget to find joy in the little things. As women, we often juggle multiple responsibilities, leaving little time for self-care and happiness. However, it's crucial to prioritize our well-being and find joy in everyday life. This subchapter explores the importance of cultivating joy and provides practical tips to help women embrace a more joyful existence.

1. Mindful Gratitude: Gratitude is a powerful tool to find joy in the present moment. Take a few minutes each day to reflect on the things you're grateful for. Whether it's a beautiful sunset, a kind gesture from a loved one, or simply having a roof over your head, acknowledging these blessings can shift your perspective and bring joy into your life.

2. Embrace Simple Pleasures: We often chase after big accomplishments and material possessions, forgetting that joy can be found in the simplest of things. Take time to appreciate a warm cup of tea, a luxurious bubble bath, or a walk in nature. These little moments can bring immense joy and contentment when we allow ourselves to fully experience them.

3. Nurture Relationships: Meaningful connections with others can bring immense joy into our lives. Invest time and energy into nurturing your relationships with family, friends, and loved ones. Engage in deep conversations, create shared experiences, and show kindness and support. These connections will not only bring joy but also provide a strong support system during challenging times.

4. Pursue Passion and Purpose: Finding joy in everyday life often involves pursuing activities that light up your soul. Discover your passions and make

time for them, whether it's painting, dancing, writing, or any other creative outlet. Engaging in activities that align with your purpose and bring you joy will enhance your overall well-being.

5. Practice Self-Care: Self-care is essential for finding joy in everyday life. Make time for activities that recharge and rejuvenate you. Whether it's practicing yoga, taking a long bath, reading a book, or meditating, prioritize self-care to replenish your energy and cultivate joy.

By incorporating these practices into your daily life, you can discover joy in even the most mundane moments. Remember, joy is not something we need to wait for; it's something we can actively cultivate and embrace in our everyday lives. Start today and embark on a journey to find joy in all aspects of your existence.

Cultivating Gratitude and Mindfulness

In today's fast-paced and hectic world, it's easy to lose sight of the things that truly matter. As women, we often put ourselves last on the priority list, sacrificing our own well-being for the sake of others. However, by cultivating gratitude and mindfulness, we can create a transformative shift in our lives and achieve holistic health and happiness.

Gratitude is a powerful tool that can completely transform our mindset and outlook on life. It allows us to shift our focus from what we lack to what we have, fostering a deep sense of appreciation for the present moment. By practicing gratitude daily, we can train our minds to seek out the positive aspects of life, even in the face of challenges. In this chapter, we will explore various techniques and exercises to cultivate gratitude, from keeping a gratitude journal to practicing random acts of kindness. You will learn how to find joy in the simple pleasures of life and develop a renewed sense of appreciation for yourself and those around you.

Mindfulness, on the other hand, is the practice of being fully present in the moment, without judgment or attachment. It allows us to slow down, tune in to our bodies, and become aware of our thoughts and emotions. Through mindfulness, we can develop a deeper understanding of ourselves and our needs, paving the way for a healthier and more balanced lifestyle. In this subchapter, we will delve into mindfulness techniques such as meditation, breathwork, and body scans. You will discover how to incorporate mindfulness into your daily routine, even in the midst of a busy schedule.

As health and wellness coaches, our mission is to assist our clients in achieving and maintaining a healthy lifestyle. By incorporating gratitude and mindfulness into our coaching practices, we can provide personalized guidance and support that goes beyond the physical aspect of wellness. We can empower women to prioritize self-care and develop a strong sense of self-love. Through gratitude and mindfulness, we can help our clients cultivate a positive mindset, reduce stress, improve sleep, and enhance overall well-being.

In this subchapter, we will not only explore the benefits of cultivating gratitude and mindfulness but also provide practical exercises and strategies to incorporate these practices into your everyday life. Embracing these principles will not only enhance your own well-being but also allow you to become a beacon of light and inspiration for those around you.

Join us on this transformative journey as we explore the power of gratitude and mindfulness in cultivating holistic health and happiness. Together, let's create a world where women prioritize their well-being and live their lives to the fullest.

Living a Purposeful and Fulfilling Life

In today's fast-paced and demanding world, it is easy to lose sight of what truly brings us joy and fulfillment. As women, we often find ourselves juggling multiple roles and responsibilities, leaving little time for self-reflection and personal growth. However, living a purposeful and fulfilling life is essential for our overall well-being and happiness.

In this subchapter, we will explore the keys to living a purposeful and fulfilling life and how it can positively impact our health and wellness. By understanding our values, setting meaningful goals, and aligning our actions with our purpose, we can experience a greater sense of fulfillment and contentment.

To begin this journey towards a purposeful life, it is crucial to reflect on our values and what truly matters to us. By identifying our core values, we can make decisions and prioritize our time based on what aligns with our authentic selves. This self-awareness allows us to create a life that is true to who we are, fostering a sense of purpose and fulfillment.

Setting meaningful goals is another vital aspect of living a purposeful life. By defining what we want to achieve and breaking it down into actionable steps, we can create a clear roadmap towards our dreams. Whether it is pursuing a career change, improving our relationships, or embarking on a personal development journey, having goals gives us direction and a sense of purpose.

However, living a purposeful life goes beyond simply setting goals; it is about taking action aligned with our purpose. It requires us to step out of our comfort zones, embrace uncertainty, and make conscious choices that bring us closer to our desired life. By taking small steps every day and making intentional decisions, we can create a life that is deeply fulfilling and meaningful.

Living a purposeful and fulfilling life has a profound impact on our health and well-being. When we are aligned with our purpose, we experience a greater sense of satisfaction, reduced stress levels, and improved mental and emotional well-being. Our relationships flourish, and we become more resilient in the face of challenges.

As health and wellness coaches, it is our mission to assist our clients in achieving and maintaining a healthy lifestyle. By guiding and supporting them in discovering their purpose and aligning their actions accordingly, we empower them to live a life of fulfillment and holistic well-being.

In conclusion, living a purposeful and fulfilling life is a transformative journey that positively impacts our health and happiness. By understanding our values, setting meaningful goals, and aligning our actions with our purpose, we can create a life that brings us joy, fulfillment, and a renewed sense of purpose. As women, let us embrace this journey and empower others to do the same, fostering holistic health and happiness in ourselves and our clients.

Conclusion: Your Journey to Holistic Health and Happiness

Congratulations, dear reader, on completing your journey through "The Wellness Woman: A Guide to Holistic Health and Happiness." As a woman, you possess an immense strength and resilience that allows you to overcome any obstacle in your path. By embarking on this journey, you have taken a significant step towards achieving and maintaining a healthy lifestyle, and we commend you for that.

Throughout this book, we have explored various aspects of holistic health and happiness, providing you with personalized guidance and support on your path. From understanding the importance of self-care and self-love to exploring the mind-body connection, we have equipped you with the tools necessary to transform your life for the better.

Remember, dear reader, that holistic health is not just about physical well-being. It encompasses every aspect of your being - mind, body, and spirit. By nurturing all these elements, you can achieve a state of balance and harmony that leads to true happiness.

As a health and wellness coach, you have the power to assist others on their own journey to holistic health. You can inspire and empower women to prioritize their well-being, guiding them towards a life of fulfillment and contentment. By sharing the knowledge and wisdom gained from this book, you can make a profound impact on the lives of those around you.

Always remember to practice what you preach. Take time for yourself, nurture your own well-being, and lead by example. By maintaining your own health and happiness, you will be better equipped to support others on their paths.

In conclusion, dear reader, we hope that this book has served as a valuable resource and guide on your journey to holistic health and happiness. Embrace the principles and practices we have discussed, and allow them to transform your life from the inside out.

Remember, your journey is ongoing. It is not the destination but the process that truly matters. Be patient with yourself, celebrate your successes, and learn from your setbacks. With dedication and perseverance, you can create a life filled with vibrant health, abundant joy, and deep fulfillment.

You are a Wellness Woman, capable of achieving anything you set your mind to. Embrace your power, honor your journey, and continue to prioritize your well-being. May your path be filled with love, light, and endless possibilities.

Wishing you a lifetime of holistic health and happiness!

With love,